The Healthy Lifestyle Diet: Clean Eating

I0417638

Eating Clean for Health and Longevity

RON KNESS

Contents

Disclaimer

This publication is for informational purposes only and is not intended as medical advice. Medical advice should always be obtained from a qualified medical professional for any health conditions or symptoms associated with them.
Every possible effort has been made in preparing and researching this material. We make no warranties with respect to the accuracy, applicability of its contents or any omissions.

See your healthcare professional before starting any diet, health or exercise program!

Introduction

Have you been considering adopting a clean eating diet? If so, kudos to you. Eating clean is a great way to take personal responsibility over your health. It also minimizes the impact that globally destructive food manufacturing processes have on the planet and its animals. In addition to your health, those are great reasons to begin eating clean today!

However, there may be a problem that is holding you back.

You might be fearful there are intricate and hard to understand rules and ideas you must follow to benefit from clean eating. You may freeze when you are standing in your grocer's produce section, trying to decide between two similar but slightly different fruits or vegetables. You may think that the complicated clean eating process is going to be too expensive or time-consuming for you and your family.

Your mind might be concerned with fitting a clean eating approach into your busy lifestyle. And you may wonder if eating clean actually tastes that good. For instance, how are you going to replace the sugar-filled junk food that you love with a healthy alternative without going into withdrawals.

These are all common thoughts people have when they consider eating clean. However, they are needless complications that do nothing but keep you from experiencing the best mental and physical health you have ever enjoyed.

Don't make the very simple process of clean eating complicated. In many cases this is a subconscious effort to justify sticking to your unhealthy refined and processed diet of fast foods and nutritionally poor food items. How easy is it to eat clean? The basic clean eating principles discussed below show you how truly simple it is.

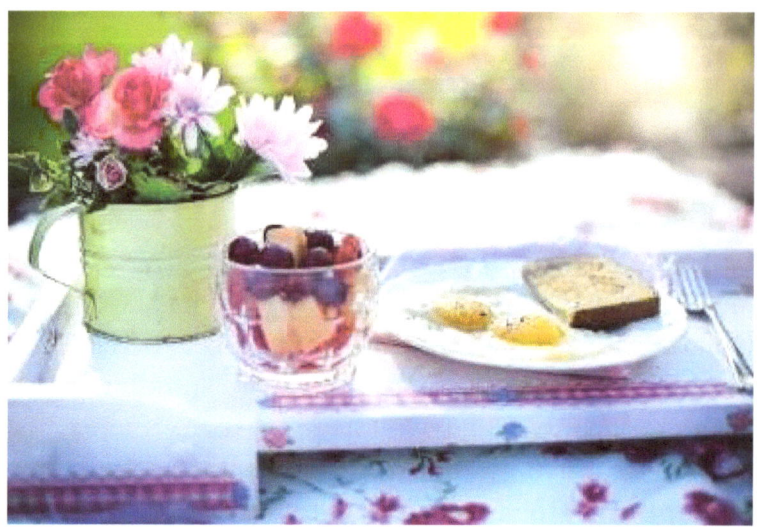

Basic Principles of Clean Eating

Do you take regular baths or showers? Of course you do! You do this to clean sweat, dead skin, dirt and debris from your skin. If you don't, you can develop skin disorders and health problems. (You will also eventually create an unpleasant odor your friends will be sure to tell you about.)

But how do you clean the inside of your body? To make the idea of clean eating simple to understand, consider it as cleaning your interior, just like bathing or showering cleans your body's exterior.

So how do you wash and clean yourself internally? You do it by limiting the amount of possibly harmful foods you eat. When you pull a carrot out of the ground and eat it, you are "eating clean". (Wash the carrot first, of course.) You are eating food as close to its natural state as you possibly can.

To think about the opposite of eating clean, imagine what happens to processed foods before they get to you. A store-bought pizza uses enriched, processed flour as its base. The veggies, cheeses and meats on the pizza have undergone injections of salt, monosodium glutamate (MSG), sugar, steroids, preservatives and other unhealthy compounds and chemical nasties.

The tomato paste used is also chock-full of unnatural and potentially harmful ingredients. This is processed food as we have come to know it, in its most nutritionally-poor form.

Obesity, heart diseases, circulatory problems and a host of other physical and mental issues are the result of a diet high in processed and refined foods.

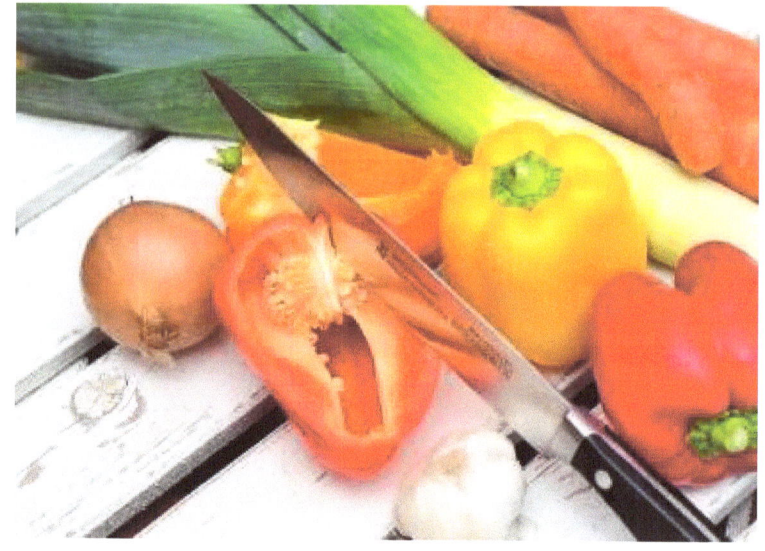

Eating clean limits, as much as possible, the amount of processed foods you eat, and focuses on whole foods – food as nature intended them to be. The reason? You can feel better, enjoy more energy, lose weight, detox your body, turn back the clock by fighting the aging process and reduce your risk of contracting a host of diseases ... simply by eating clean.

The Simple Basics of Clean Eating

Eat more whole foods - Whole foods are very close to their original state. Sure, apples and oranges went through some type of process to get from a farm or orchard and to your grocer. Better yet, if you live close to an orchard, go pick fruit directly off the trees. It doesn't get any more fresh than that!

Regardless if you pick it yourself or buy it already picked, the fruit has enjoyed minimal human intrusion compared to processed foods. Whole fruits and vegetables, grass-fed, free-range meat products, unsalted seeds and nuts, and whole grains, along with organic are what you want to focus on eating here.

Eat fewer processed foods - This is easier to do than you may think. If the food you are about to eat comes in a wrapper or package, it has been processed. Check the ingredients label. Some foods that are wrapped up or packaged have minimal processing. Most do not. By just avoiding anything in a wrapper, you will drastically and simply limit your intake of processed and refined foods and eat more clean ... just from that one change!

Eat more frequently - The Standard American Diet (appropriately shortened to SAD) is also enjoyed in most modern countries and cultures. I don't know that it is necessarily a good thing.

It includes eating 3 meals a day, huge portions and guaranteed to minimize your overall wellness and maximize poor health. Instead spread your total daily eating over 5 or 6 smaller sessions. Eat smaller quantities, and eat every 2 or 3 hours, either a meal or snack, however your total calories should remain the same that is appropriate for your age, weight and exercise level. Eating this way keeps your metabolism super-charged because it always has food available, and your internal processes working properly.

Prepare your own meals - The best way to eat clean is to know exactly what goes into the food you eat. Eating away from home means you are playing Russian roulette with your diet. Cook your own meals using whole food and ingredients and there is no mystery as far as what you are eating.

Eat balanced meals and snacks – Make sure you are getting carbohydrates, proteins and healthy fats with any meal or snack. This combination makes you feel full longer. It also reduces your urges for unhealthy junk and processed foods.

Stop killing yourself by eating refined sugar - Did you know that sugar creates a reaction in your brain similar to that of a drug addiction, much like heroin? Refined, processed sugar is regarded by most health officials and doctors as the major cause for obesity today. This leads to circulatory, respiratory and cardiovascular problems, an increased risk of contracting diabetes, and a host of mental and physical health issues. The empty calories in sugar do absolutely nothing positive for your body. Natural sweeteners (fructose) are found in fruits and vegetables, and can easily replace potentially deadly refined sugar, or worse yet artificial sweeteners.

Constantly remind yourself of the above 6 traits of clean eating. If you simply wrote the above 6 tips on a piece of paper and referred to it every time you shopped for groceries, you and your family could benefit from the wonderful health properties of clean eating without making the process more complicated than it actually is or needs to be.

In our introduction, we covered some of the common concerns about clean eating. These included how to eat clean without breaking the bank, and finding the time to eat clean for the busy, modern-day family. You may also wonder how to make your clean meals delicious and tasty, and how to make mouthwatering sweets and treats without straying from your clean eating plans. Each of those important concerns is covered in detail below.

How to Eat Clean on a Budget

A principal concern about clean eating is how physically clean your foods are. Non-organic farmers use pesticides and other chemicals to treat their fields of fruits and vegetables. Does this mean you have to eat nothing but expensive organic food to eat clean?

Absolutely not.

In the United States and the United Kingdom, foods and vegetables that make it to your grocer's shelves are fine for human consumption. The same is true in other modernized societies. The amount of contaminants or chemicals present is within the accepted levels. **Your health won't suffer appreciably if you choose "regular" foods over their organic cousins.**

You should also remember that you **don't need to equip your kitchen with expensive appliances** to eat clean. A food processor does make creating pastes, purees and mixes easier to prepare, but it is not required.

You will probably find that eating clean **can actually be less expensive** than your current dietary approach. You can **buy raw whole foods in bulk** to save money. You can shop, slice, dice and prepare individual food items and entire meals in advance, and store serving sizes in your refrigerator and freezer.

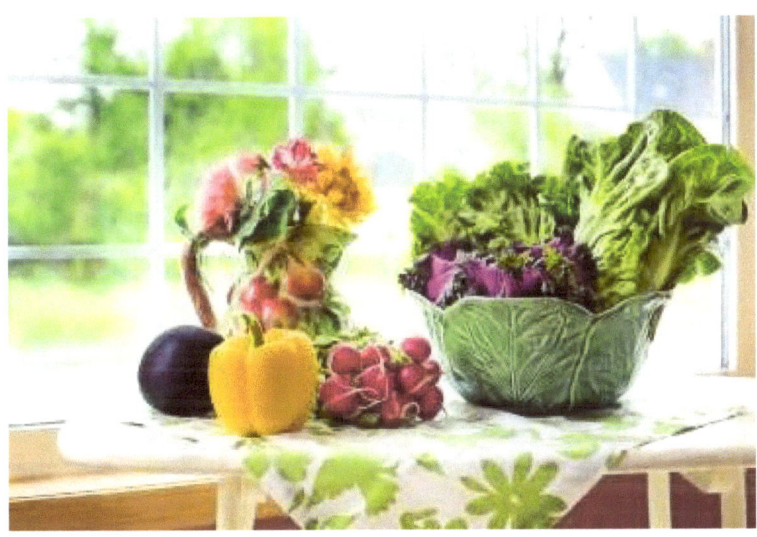

Another monetary expense which drops drastically when you adopt a clean eating attitude (and one most people don't think about) is **your annual medical expenses.** There is no arguing that clean eating leads to better health than eating processed and refined foods. Your wallet or pocketbook is going to appreciate the substantial drop in medical bills that clean eating delivers.

Shop for in-season produce whenever you can. As a benefit, vegetables and fruits are at the height of their flavor and nutrition when they are in season. Strawberries, peaches, cherries and melons are excellent values in the summer months.

Also, don't forget that inexpensive **frozen fruits and vegetables are sometimes more nutritious** than the non-frozen choices in the produce section. These foods go immediately from a farm to a packaging company where they are flash frozen. They are at the peak of ripeness. This limits the amount of time that produce has to lose nutrients and minerals due to exposure to the air.

Focus on store brand frozen fruits and vegetables for the biggest savings. And frozen makes a great alternative when fresh in not in season.

Spice It Up! Keeping Your Meals Tasty

Salt and pepper are the two predominant spices found in modern-day kitchens. Fresh, cracked black pepper is very healthy for you. It also is an excellent and versatile spice. Salt, on the other hand, can be downright deadly. Most humans living in a developed society get plenty of salt in their diet. This means any additional salt can cause health problems.

Fortunately, there are dozens of herbs and spices that naturally deliver a wide range of wonderful flavors.

Basil – This spicy herb is native to tropical Asia. It is perfect for flavoring pork, lamb, poultry and tomato-based dishes. Add basil closer to the end of the cooking process, since its oils are highly volatile. This allows you to retain the most flavor possible from this natural herb.

Turmeric – The powerful, bitter flavor of turmeric masks cancer fighting properties. This is considered one of the healthiest spices found anywhere. It gives food an unmistakable yellow tint. Also known as an effective spice for controlling your weight, turmeric is perfect with egg salad, rice dishes, beans and salads.

Cinnamon – Cinnamon comes from the bark of a tropical evergreen tree. It is at home in desserts and puddings, as well as cakes, pies and other baked goods.

Medical research shows that cinnamon is full of healthy antioxidants, has wonderful anti-inflammatory properties and may reduce your risk of contracting heart disease.

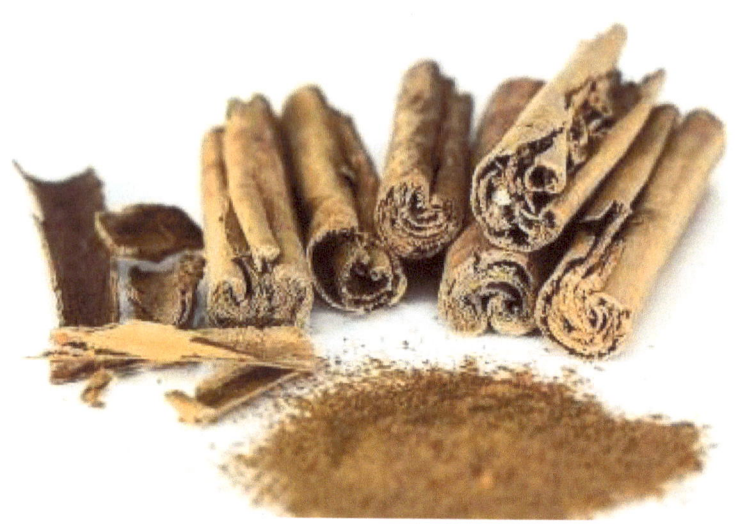

Parsley – Easily the most popular herb in the world, parsley is also considered one of the healthiest foods on the planet. Parsley delivers vitamin C, B12, vitamin K and vitamin A. It helps you flush excess fluid from your body, heals your nervous system, regulates a healthy blood pressure and may reduce hair loss when massaged into the scalp! This versatile superfood has a vibrant, fresh taste that complements seafood, pasta, soups and vegetables.

Garlic – This heart-healthy bulb delivers a pungent and hot sweetness. Its uses for flavoring are pretty limitless in the kitchen, so experiment freely.

Mint – This aromatic herb delivers a sweet, warm flavor with a slightly cool aftertaste. It is ideally suited for teas and other beverages, jellies and syrups.

Nutmeg – Myristica fragrans, more commonly known as nutmeg, comes from an evergreen tree too – similar to cinnamon. The nutmeg seed produces a powder that is sweet and delicate in flavor.

Marjoram, oregano, sage, rosemary, thyme, cloves, cumin, cayenne pepper, cilantro, ginger, mace, paprika and sage round out the herbs and spices that can flavor up a multitude of meals.

Clean Eating for Busy Families

If you and your family are extremely busy (as most are today), welcome to the club. Most modern families are starved for time on a daily basis. However, you should not opt for the fast food lane instead of clean eating simply because you have a hectic lifestyle.

Some households cook a week's worth of meals for their family as soon as they get home from their weekly grocery shopping. Taking one day per week to shop and cook can make the other six days seem like a breeze.

If you are the chief cook (and bottle washer), enlist the help of other family members in the kitchen. If your kids help you cook healthy meals from nutritious whole foods, they're more likely to actually eat the food they make and stay with eating healthy once they leave the house. It is a life skill all kids should know!

Take baby steps by slowly incorporating clean eating into your current dietary approach. Take salt and refined sugar out of your pantry and off of your table. Replace them with healthy herbs and spices, some of the ones we just mentioned in the last section. This makes it quick and easy to make smart clean eating choices.

Remind your family exactly why you are adopting a clean eating lifestyle. Reward your children when they choose a clean meal over a processed one. Prepackage clean snacks for your child's lunchbox and your workplace.

Get in the daily habit of making clean eating choices, and your busy lifestyle won't get in the way of the healthy rewards you are looking for.

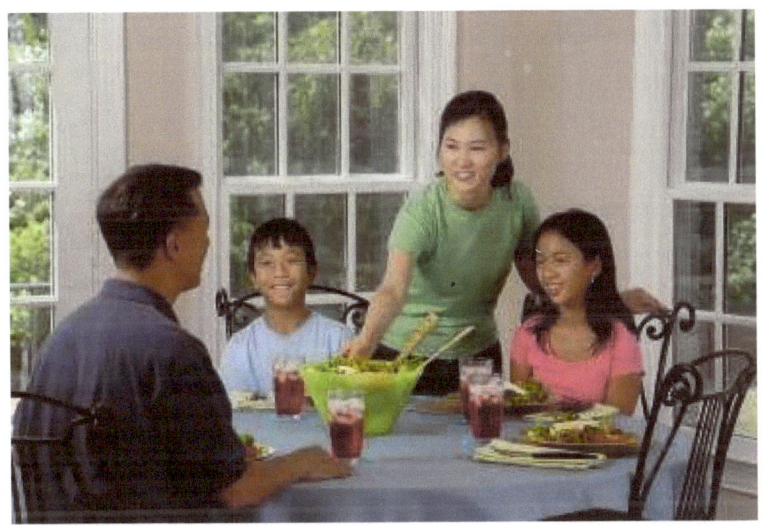

Clean Food Hacks for Baking and Sweet Treats

Refined sugar is a scrumptious ingredient found in a lot of sweet treats and baked goods. As mentioned earlier, it is also potentially deadly. You probably unwittingly get way too much sugar in your currently processed and fast food diet because of added sugar. Consider this:

The World Health Organization (WHO) and American Heart Association recommend between 6 teaspoons (women) and 9 teaspoons (men) as a daily dietary maximum. The problem is that an average beverage, like a 12-ounce soda or 8-ounce energy drink can deliver all of the sugar you should ingest in an entire day in just one drink!

This is why switching to clean foods, like whole foods, is so important. Foods and drinks that you never thought contained sugar are packed full of it. This is because sugar is a cheap preservative and sweetener.

If you know you are addicted to sugar, don't worry. Clean eating provides natural sweeteners to replace your unhealthy addiction. Start replacing sugar with the following 5 natural foods today and your unhealthy cravings will be satisfied with naturally healthy foods.

1 - Pumpkin - Mashed or puréed pumpkin is more versatile in the kitchen than you may imagine. Just 1/2 cup of pumpkin replaces 2 eggs, 2 tablespoons of sugar and 1/2 cup of oil in just about any recipe. It is extremely high in healthy dietary fiber, so your sweets and treats make you feel full longer.

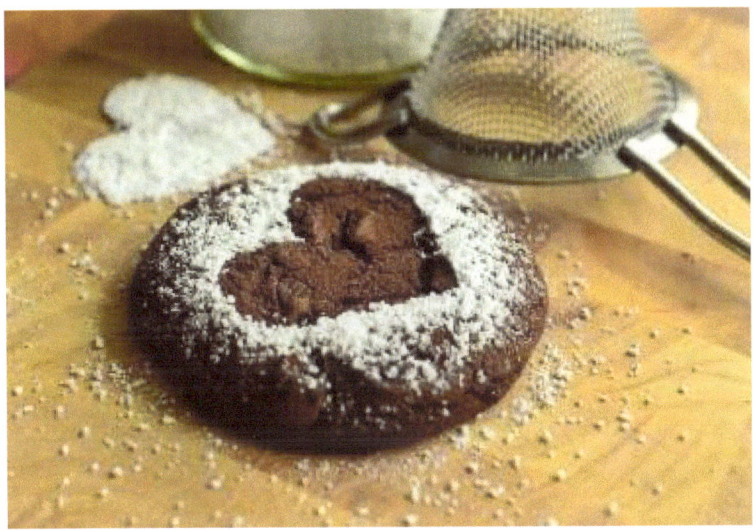

2 - Sweet potato - Just like the previous clean food on this list, sweet potatoes are excellent natural sweeteners. Use them to create healthy and delicious muffins, breads and cookies. Canned sweet potato is convenient, just make sure you check your food label to ensure no added sugar is present.

3 - Dried fruit - Raisins, dates, figs, apricots and berries all have very unique and noticeable flavors. You can soak dried fruit before you chop or puree it for a sweet paste that you can use in a number of recipes. Be forewarned, these foods are high in natural sugar, so use them in limited quality.

4 - Applesauce - This clean eating ingredient only qualifies as such when you choose the unsweetened version. This is a clean eating standby for replacing oil and sugar in many recipes. Consider a 1 to 1 quantity exchange for sugar. You may also consider apple chunks and apple butter, as long as they have no sugar added.

5 - Spices - Some spices offer a naturally sweet flavor (see the previous section on **Spice It Up! How to Keep Your Clean Meals Tasty**. Nutmeg, cloves, cinnamon, ginger and cardamom are considered sweet spices. Combine them with any of the suggested sugar alternatives above for a savory, sweet combination.

Clean Eating for Losing Weight

In the mid-1800s, Justus Von Liebig introduced chemicals to farming. He found that if correct levels of nitrogen, potassium and phosphorus were maintained in soil, crop yields were positively affected. Almost as soon as that German chemist began preaching his chemical-industrial agriculture beliefs, concerns about the effect on humans was raised.

Although clean eating has exploded in popularity over the last 20 years, it seems there were people worried about the effect of chemicals on the foods we eat ever since Von Liebig introduced fertilizer to agriculture.

It just makes sense to inspect and respect the foods we put into our bodies. The old saying that you are what you eat is definitely true. Mankind has never been more obese, sickly and unhealthy than it is today. It is no wonder, since the processed foods we eat are bloated with man-made chemicals, artificial ingredients and addictive compounds, which our bodies have no idea how to process so it gets stored as fat, that we experience unhealthy consequences usually in the form of overweight and obesity.

Because of this health concern of epidemic proportions, weight loss programs and fad diets are selling better than ever. If the proponents of these "miracle diets" were selling and telling the truth, why are we still fat, overweight and out of shape?

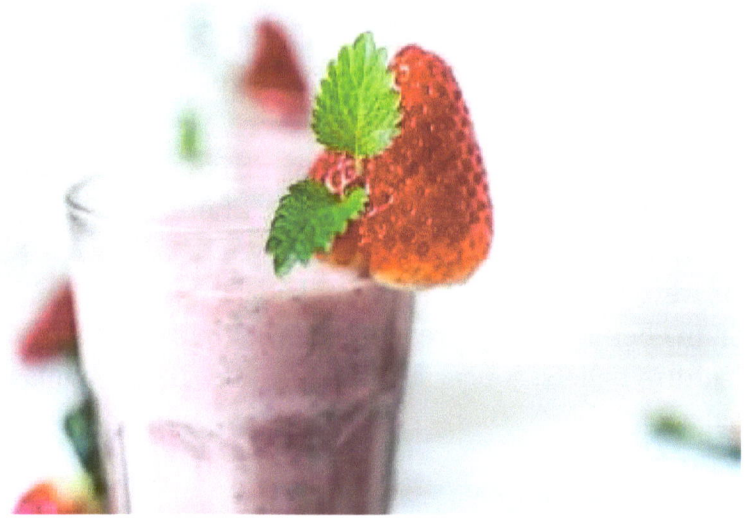

The answer is simple.

Most diets do not address your nutritional needs. Many of them will indeed help you lose weight quickly. But since most fad diets are nutritionally poor and unsustainable over the long-term, you end up reverting back to eating junk food and replacing the weight you lost, and then some.

This is why clean eating has become increasingly popular for losing weight. Eating clean is perfectly suited to fat burning and healthy body weight regulation because of one simple reason ...

... Clean Eating Provides All the Nutrition You Need

Clean eating is nothing more than making the decision to eat whole, unprocessed foods rather than refined and processed foods. That's it. There are no calories to count and no measurements to make.

You stock your refrigerator, freezer and pantry with healthy, whole fruits, vegetables, whole grains, grass-fed meats, lean poultry, beans, peas and legumes. When you are hungry, you eat.

That is how simple and basic clean eating is.

Why is it so good for losing weight, making you healthy, fighting disease and providing plenty of energy? Because the components of a clean eating lifestyle provide all the minerals and nutrition you need for your body to work properly.

This means if you are overweight, or even obese, from years of eating processed food which is slowly killing you, changing to a clean eating program will naturally and effortlessly return you to your healthy body weight and helps you stay there. No fancy diet needed!

Since your body is getting all the nutrition it needs, you don't go on unhealthy eating binges. You feel full all day long when you eat clean food 5 or 6 times a day. So you don't wind up ordering late night delivery pizza and knocking your diet plans out of whack. You feel healthy, and since you are only eating nutritious food, your body starts to shed any unnecessary body fat.

Your body gets what it wants, and you get what you want. A win/win situation for both of you!

The result is you reaching and maintaining your natural, healthy body weight. It might not be the size 2 you were hoping for, but it is a size and weight that is comfortable for your body composition.

Your size 2 goal was probably unrealistic anyway and even if you had gotten there, you would not have stayed at that size over the long-term. Extra bonuses are a reduced risk of heart disease, diabetes and other illnesses, as well as plenty of natural energy and a great feeling of accomplishment. The compliments you get from your friends, family, coworkers and significant other aren't bad either.

Clean eating also builds more muscle than a diet rich in processed and refined foods. Why is this important if you are looking to lose weight? Because the more muscle you have, the more fat you burn.

A lean, muscular body needs more energy than an overweight, out of shape person. The reason why your body stores fat is as an energy source. So when you eat clean, you naturally build more muscle, which in turn effortlessly increases the amount of fat you burn.

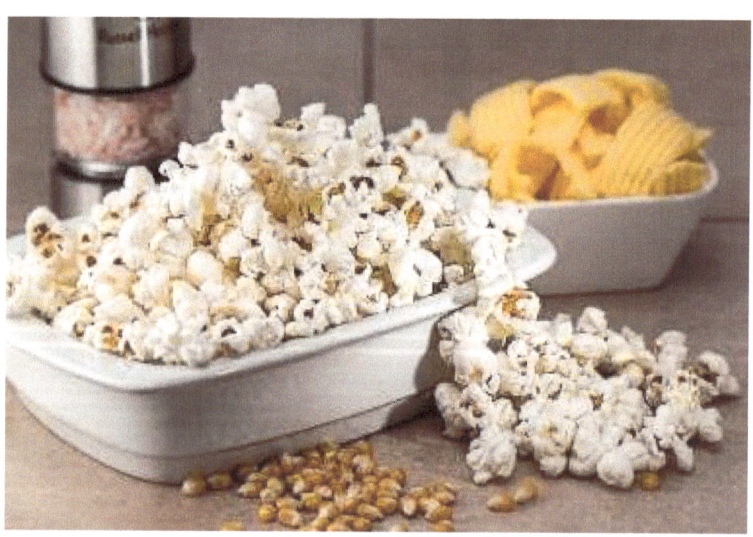

Clean vs Dirty Food Calories - What's the Difference?

Have you ever heard anyone talk about "empty calories". What they are referring to are the (dirty) calories contained in food that has little nutritional value.

Sugar is an excellent example.

You get all the sugar you need, healthy sugar, from natural, unprocessed foods. Too much sugar is not a good thing, however. If you drink too much water, it will simply and harmlessly flush out of your body. Sugar does not work the same way. Excess sugar is stored as fat in your body. It has little to no nutritional value, but does have a calorie load.

This means if you eat foods with a lot of sugar, you are delivering little nutrition to your body, but lots of calories.

Consider these "dirty calories" since they are unhealthy for you. If you eat 2,000 dirty calories, calories with very little nutritional value, your brain will still send out hunger signals. This is because even though you may have consumed the proper amount of calories for the day, your body did not receive any nutrition.

This is why you are often hungry after gorging on fast food and processed food. Your body did not get the minerals, and vitamins, enzymes and healthy phytonutrients it needs to function properly. So you find yourself hungry, even though you have just ingested a ton of food. Since sugar and other chemicals intentionally put in the processed food are very addictive, what food do you think you reach for when you experience these hunger pangs?

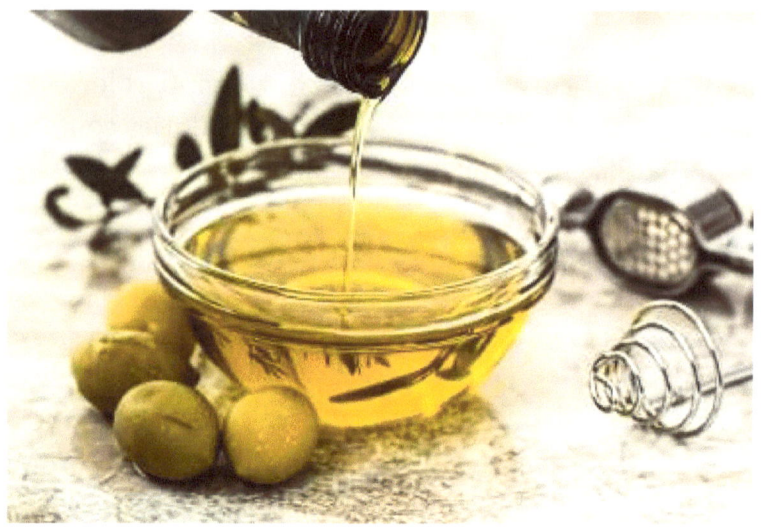

You of course reach for the same nutritionally poor processed and refined foods that caused this problem in the first place.

The result is you continue to pack on the pounds, since sugar, trans fat and other additives and preservatives in processed food are stored as fat in your body.

This is why you have to be careful about your choice of calories. It is also another reason why clean eating is so good for burning fat, and for healthy body weight regulation. Clean foods like vegetables, fiber, whole grains and fruits are what nutritionists call "nutrient dense" foods. Even small amounts of those foods are loaded with the nutrients and minerals your body needs. However, they do not carry near the calorie count that dirty foods do.

For example, just **1 tablespoon of standard table sugar packs in about 48 calories.** On the other hand, **an entire cup of broccoli has just 31 calories!**

Unfortunately, sugar does not make you feel full. It also delivers no significant nutrition. So you can eat it all day long and still feel hungry.

One cup of broccoli delivers 2.4 g of dietary fiber. Fiber takes longer to process in your digestive tract than simple carbohydrates like sugar. This means you feel full longer, eat less during the day, and that single cup of broccoli also offers 2.57 g of protein, 0.34 g of healthy fat and 6.04 g of carbohydrates.

Examples of Dirty and Clean Calories

Dirty calories are found in baked goods, any food with added sugar, processed, refined foods and fast foods. Dirty calories come from solid fats and or added sugars. Sodas, fruit drinks, beer, ice cream, fried foods, margarine and butter, doughnuts, deli meats, cake and cookies are all examples of foods packed full of dirty calories.

On the other hand, clean calories are found in whole foods. Whole foods are those foods which are minimally processed, or not processed at all. They take the shortest trip from the farm to your plate. They are not loaded with additives, preservatives, artificial ingredients, sugar, salt, MSG and other nutritional nightmares. Lean cuts of grass-fed beef, skinless, boneless, organic chicken, wild caught salmon, apples, beans, whole grains, romaine lettuce and any fresh, unprocessed fruits and vegetables are delicious examples of clean calories.

Eating Clean in a Way That Works for You

You may have noticed by now that a lot of the food you eat on a daily basis is "dirty". If you are an average human being living in a modern society, you are also not eating near the amounts of clean foods that you should be. This is a double-edged sword that is cutting you wrong in two ways.

You may also think it is going to be tough for you to give up all of the harmful foods you love.

Don't worry, you can eat clean in a way that is uniquely yours. Remember the following tips, and you will find yourself eating more clean food, less dirty food, and doing so without a lot of mental stress and aggravation.

Eating clean is not a zero-sum game. Clean eating does not have to be an all or nothing scenario – while ideal, it is not sustainable; after all we are all human and prone to make mistakes now and then. Eating is no different.

If you still desire less than healthy foods from time to time, enjoy a serving or two. Just don't let dirty eating dominate your dietary plans.

Take it slow to begin with. You may have been eating dirty food your entire life. Your body could have developed powerful addictions to foods like salt and sugar. This will take time to turn around. Take baby steps at first, slowly integrating clean foods into your diet, adding more and more over time.

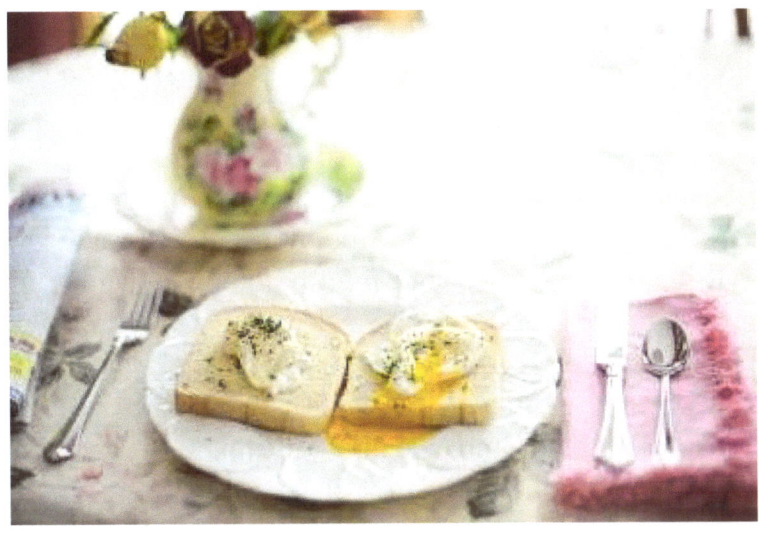

Aim for the process and not the weight loss. If you begin eating clean, the pounds will come off. You don't have to count them and measure them. Yes, it is powerfully motivating to jump on that scale and see you have lost 5 pounds. Just remember your day-to-day clean eating actions are what makes weight loss possible.

Don't forget to eat. A lot of diet plans virtually starve you. You don't have to feel starved when you eat clean. These foods are so nutritionally rich, while still delivering a relatively low calorie load, that you can eat whenever you're hungry without worrying about packing on body fat and gaining tons of weight. Some whole foods are negative calorie sum meaning it takes more calories to process then they contain.

High-fiber foods make you feel full longer. They also support a healthy digestive system. Broccoli, whole-grains, lentils and beans, berries, avocados, pears, almonds, artichoke and sweet potatoes are just a few examples of high-fiber whole foods.

Because they take longer to digest, you won't have the hunger cravings and end up eating something not good for you.

Write down what you eat ... every bite. It is easy to underestimate how much dirty food you eat. Keep a record of everything that goes into your mouth, food and drinks, and you will find it easier to stick to a clean eating regimen once you have a written record. Most people far underestimate how much they eat in terms of calories, unhealthy fats, salt and sugar. Some have no clue at all or even know how much they should be eating in the first place.

11 Healthy Clean Snack Ideas

Clean eating for weight loss means taking snack time seriously. You can wreck your plans quickly, and pack on the pounds, if your snacks and treats are dirty instead of clean. The following 11 healthy and clean snack ideas will keep you headed in the right direction with your weight loss efforts.

Make fruit and veggie kebabs. Crisp, cool, diced fruit on a shish-kebab makes a fun and fiber-filled treat for kids and adults in the summer. Shish-kebabs with your favorite vegetables cooked over the backyard grill and drizzled with coconut oil are delicious as well.

Diced apple chunks dipped in guacamole are as healthy and filling as they are delicious. Either make your own guacamole at home, or be sure to read the ingredients label to make sure there are no unhealthy additives present.

Roast your favorite nuts. Unsalted walnuts, almonds and pecans can be roasted with a light coating of coconut or olive oil. Add your favorite herbs and spices for a wonderfully nutritious snack which is extremely portable and enjoys a long shelf life.

Apple slices brushed with olive oil and baked until crisp provide a healthy replacement for potato chips.

Frozen berries. This is a healthy and cool treat in the summer. You can also coat your favorite berries in low-fat, Greek yogurt and place on a baking sheet in your freezer for 2 hours for a unique taste treat.

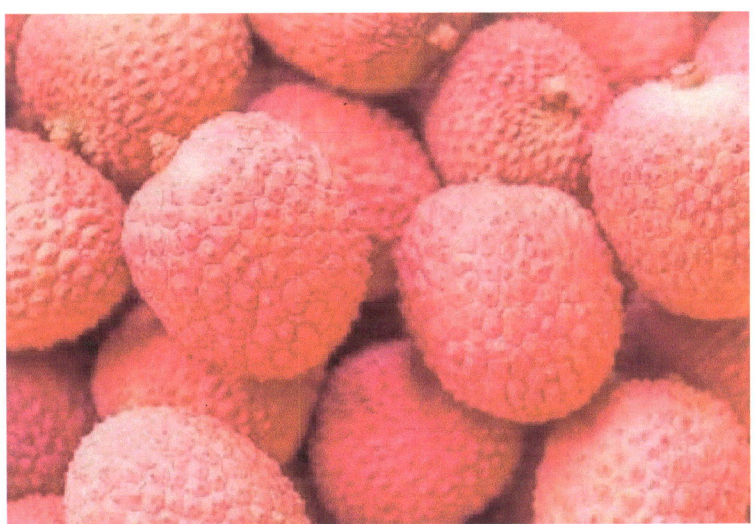

Fresh mashed avocado on whole-grain toast is a quick and easy snack that you can top with your favorite herbs and spices.

Fresh fruit is a simple and extremely healthy clean eating snack. Grab a banana, apple or handful of strawberries instead of reaching for a processed snack.

Boil a dozen eggs and keep them in your fridge for a yummy and nutritious quick snack. Eggs contain what nutrition experts call the perfect protein.

Leftovers! Why not have a semi-serving of whatever clean eating entrée that is left over in your refrigerator? This minimizes waste and requires no preparation.

Fruit salad is quick and easy to make, and the different textures and flavors of your favorite fruits makes for a delicious treat.

Ants on a log. Stuff celery sticks with organic peanut butter, hummus and guacamole. Top with raisins.

Clean Eating During Pregnancy

Are you or someone you know expecting? If so, congratulations are in order. This is an exciting and miraculous period of time, for the mom-to-be as well as any family members and friends. A new addition, whether it is the first or the fifth, means some traditional pregnancy traits and characteristics are soon to appear.

For instance, it is well-known that pregnant women often crave very odd combinations of foods. This is usually because there is some nutritional imbalance at work. A woman "with child" doesn't suddenly desire chocolate ice cream, sardines and peanut butter simply because she has never tried that gastrointestinal delight before. There is a nutritional need screaming to be filled.

That is where clean eating can help.

If you are unfamiliar with what "eating clean" entails, it is rather simple. You restrict refined and processed foods, and eat whole foods instead. Whole foods are foods that are close to their natural state. They are minimally refined and processed, free from unnecessary additives, preservatives and artificial ingredients, making them a better choice for your baby.

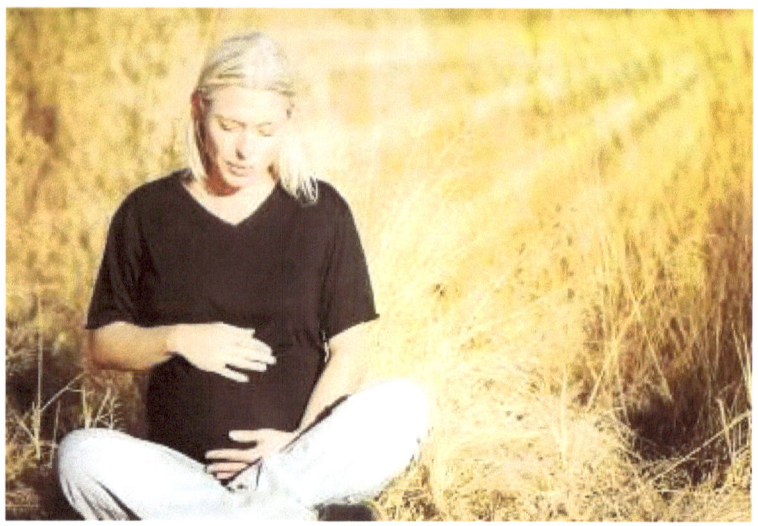

This means clean eating includes fresh vegetables, fruits and whole grains. Beans, berries, unsalted nuts and grass-fed meats are acceptable as well. If you were eating clean before becoming pregnant, very few changes will have to be made3 to your diet.

This nutritional profile delivers everything a human being needs for optimal health. It also limits the refined sugar, salt, white flour, trans fats, MSG and other harmful ingredients that plague the modern day diet.

So, what considerations does a pregnant woman need to make if she is planning on eating clean for better health, for both her and her unborn child?

First off, always follow your doctor's advice. He or she is a trained medical professional that has "seen it all before" concerning pregnancies. First and foremost, listen to your doctor. You and your child's best interests are at the heart of all the decisions your doctor makes. So pay heed.

Aside from supplements and some other dietary considerations we will cover later, your doctor will probably applaud your clean eating efforts.

Modern medicine understands the incredible changes your body goes through during pregnancy. Because of this, we now know there are certain chemical imbalances which must be corrected quickly, as well as other nutritional concerns which need to be met. Let's take a look at some typical dietary concerns many pregnant women need to address.

Understanding Standard Pregnancy Dietary Precautions

A pregnant woman's body must provide for her own health needs, as well as those of her unborn child. This is why it is ideal for all women of childbearing age to constantly eat a smart and healthy diet. Clean eating can help you do that.

However, once you become pregnant, your nutritional needs change drastically. Not necessarily in the kind of food if you are eating clean already, but the amount of food or more directly the number of calories consumed.

For example, you will need to **increase your diet by approximately 300 calories a day starting with your second trimester.** This needs to include 60 to 80 grams of protein each and every day. That high-protein intake needs to account for approximately 20% to 25% of your daily calories.

Clean eating involves plenty of healthy, whole foods which are protein-rich. Eggs, grass-fed beef, beans, boneless and skinless chicken breast and cold water fish are excellent sources of protein which allow you to adhere to a clean eating diet.

You also need to increase your intake of complex carbohydrates. Simple carbohydrates and starches, found in white bread, pretzels and cookies, potato chips and sugar, do not deliver the nutritional punch that complex carbs do. Once again clean eating arrives on the scene with an answer.

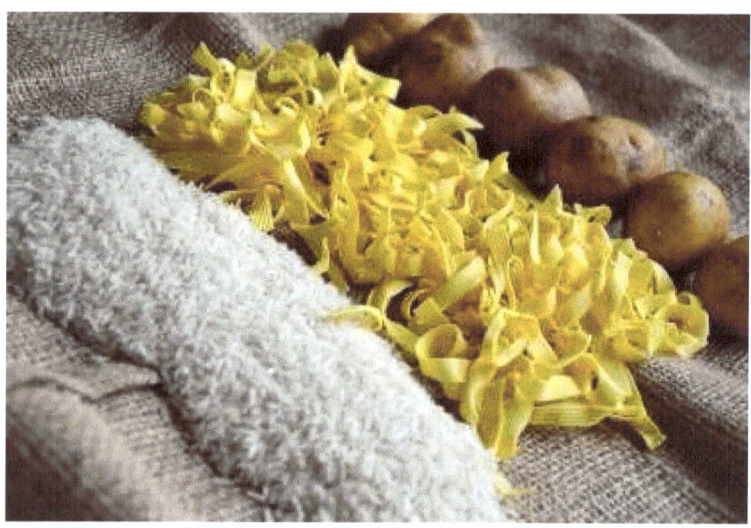

Pregnant woman can benefit from complex carbs found in whole foods like whole-grain breads and pastas, legumes, beans and vegetables.

Constipation is something pregnant women sometimes develop. Because of the complex process their body is going through, poor diet can lead to difficulty having bowel movements.

Eating plenty of whole foods which include leafy greens like kale and cabbage, and full of dietary fiber such as broccoli and peas, ensures that constipation is not an issue.

Most doctors will recommend a **balanced diet** full of fruits, vegetables, whole grains, protein-rich non-processed foods and dairy products for pregnant women. It just so happens that those are all foods which make up a clean eating lifestyle. (Clean eating usually focuses on low-fat dairy products).

Calcium is needed for proper formation of your child's teeth and bones. Doctors recommend at least 1,000 mg per day while you are pregnant. This mineral can be found in abundance in green, leafy vegetables.

Women are naturally prone to iron deficiencies. You need a full 27 mg a day while you are pregnant. Fish, lean cuts of poultry, dried fruits and liver are excellent clean eating sources of iron.

Of course, a healthy pregnancy and birth depend on a properly hydrated body. Water is the simplest one-ingredient beverage in the clean eating plan. Pregnant or not, women (and men and children) should be drinking plenty of water every day.

Why a Healthy Pregnancy Diet Is Important for Baby

Giving your child the best start at life is first and foremost in your mind. You can do this by following the dietary advice mentioned above as far as protein, iron, complex carbohydrates and other nutritional factors are concerned.

This is crucial because your child is growing at an incredibly rapid rate physiologically and mentally during your pregnancy.

The March of Dimes reports that a full 70% of all neural tube defects can be avoided entirely by proper pregnancy nutrition. Neural tube defects occur when you do not get enough folic acid during your pregnancy. Folic acid is important to create the extra blood you and your unborn child need during pregnancy.

Spinach, romaine lettuce, broccoli and kale are very rich in folic acid. Simply eating enough of those vegetables can ensure you get enough of this important acid during pregnancy.

A healthy pregnancy diet also means avoiding certain foods.

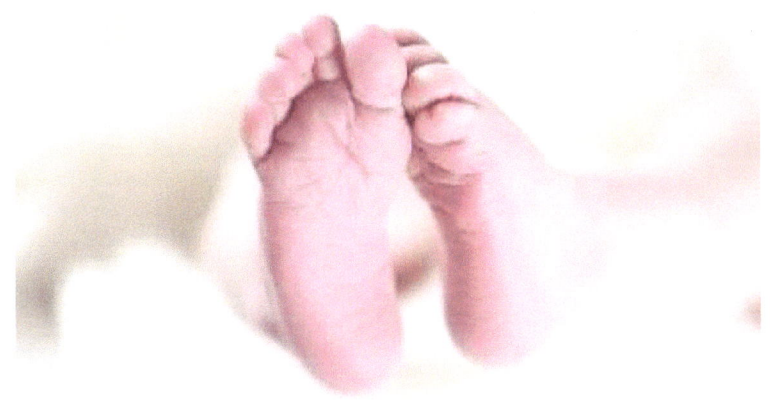

It is commonly known that alcohol should be avoided entirely during pregnancy. Alcohol from beer, wine and adult beverages can pass immediately to your unborn child through your umbilical cord. Heavy alcohol use during pregnancy is linked to an increased chance that your child will be born with fetal alcohol spectrum disorders. This can cause physical and mental as well as behavioral difficulties.

A healthy pregnancy diet is also important for your child's vision. Eating too much raw meat during pregnancy can infect your child with Toxoplasma. This can lead to blindness later in life, and means avoiding sushi, carpaccio, undercooked shellfish along with undercooked meats and poultry during your pregnancy.

You should also entirely avoid raw or undercooked eggs. This can include runny or poached eggs, and foods like cookie dough or cake batter, hollandaise sauce and homemade ice cream. Those foods can increase the risk of food poisoning in a pregnant woman, passing vision and other health problems along to your child.

Eat plenty of whole grains and vegetables while you are pregnant. Feast on fresh fruits, lean, grass-fed beef and poultry, and fish like salmon and mackerel. Whole grains, legumes, peas and beans will also give your baby the best chance at a healthy pregnancy and childhood.

Avoiding Unhealthy Weight Gain During Pregnancy

The number one complaint of pregnant women is often the added weight they put on. This is a chief concern that your doctor will discuss with you as well. Eating a clean diet during pregnancy, along with whatever vitamin and mineral supplements your doctor prescribes, is ideal for keeping your weight gain in check.

The American College of Obstetricians and Gynecologists has defined the "normal" weight gain for a healthy pregnancy. **If you gain between 25 and 35 pounds while you are pregnant, this is considered an average and acceptable amount.** Obviously, your pre-pregnancy weight and physical condition must be considered.

If you weighed 110 pounds before getting pregnant, and find yourself 40 pounds overweight during pregnancy, this is going to be a problem. Alternately, there are cases of obese women who didn't realize they were pregnant until right before they gave birth.

Sticking to a diet full of whole grains, fruits and vegetables, while getting plenty of protein and complex carbohydrates, can help pregnant women keep from gaining an unhealthy amount of weight.

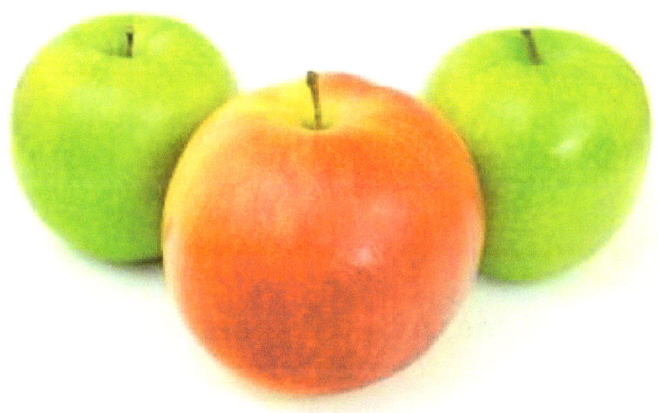

Your doctor will monitor your weight gain. Pregnancy is a very structured process these days. Your doctor will let you know when you are under or overweight for someone your size, age and stage of pregnancy. Discuss with your doctor what clean eating foods would be recommended to gain or lose the weight they suggest.

Be careful looking at just your weight as a simple number though.

You will gain a lot of water weight when you are pregnant. Water does not provide the nutritional components you and your unborn child need for a healthy pregnancy and birth.

This is why a constant monitoring of your mineral and nutrient profile by your doctor is extremely important so your clean eating plan can provide for a healthy pregnancy, while keeping you at an ideal weight.

5 Additional Healthy Pregnancy Diet Tips

1 - Don't Obsess over Dietary Perfection. Your mental health is just as important as your physical health where your baby is concerned. If you're constantly stressed out, research shows that can negatively affect your child's development.

2 - Eat 5 or 6 Times A Day. You are going to be eating a lot. It is better to eat periodically throughout the day, so your body can process all that extra food. This is easier on you, and better for your unborn child.

3 - Start Eating Smart Before You Get Pregnant. If you eat a poor diet, it is going to be tough to immediately change to a healthy one when you become pregnant. Begin eating clean today if you are of childbearing age.

4 - Never Skip Breakfast. This is important in general, and specifically what you are pregnant. If you are experiencing morning sickness, at least eat some whole-grain toast. Then eat more later in the morning.

5 - Eat 12 to 16 Ounces of Fish or Shellfish Each Week. A serving of fish approximately the size of a deck of playing cards is 3 ounces. Avoid shark, tile fish and swordfish because of possibly high levels of mercury.

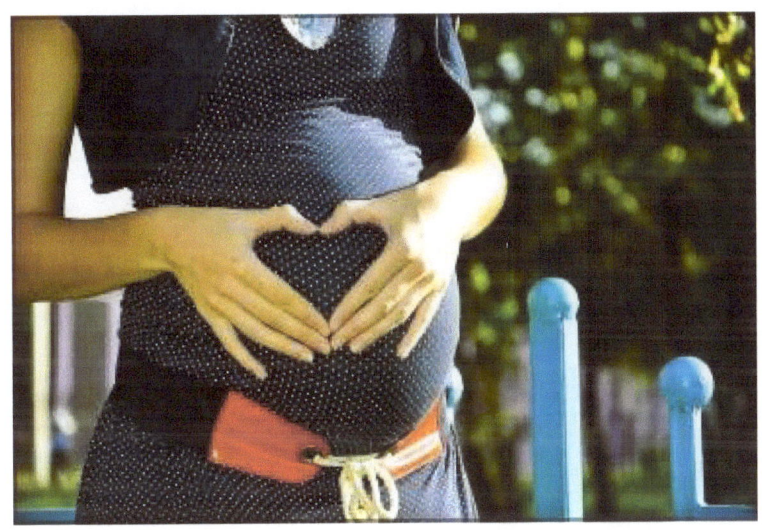

Final Thoughts

Eating clean is only complicated and difficult if you make it that way. Everything that you get in life which is worth achieving or accomplishing is going to depend on the choices that you make. Clean eating versus eating a lot of processed foods means living a longer, happier and healthier life.

Is that something you want? Then make the smart choice.

Begin practicing the 6 simple basics for clean eating discussed earlier. Write those 6 characteristics of healthy clean eating on a notepad you keep it with you when you make your grocery shopping lists. Download any of the many clean eating apps available for your preferred mobile device.

This makes it very simple to make the right decisions when you are shopping for the food your family is going to eat.

Remember, a sugar addiction took time to develop. It may take some time to beat as well. Research shows that 3 to 4 weeks of a diet absent of refined sugar is all it takes most people to kick their sugar habit. Besides, there are plenty of natural sweeteners found in whole foods like fruits and vegetables. This makes it easy to bake desserts, snacks and treats that satisfy your sweet tooth while sticking to a clean eating profile.

You now know that clean eating can actually be less expensive than your current eating habits (and a whole lot healthier!). And you now know some tips you can use to integrate clean eating as a part of a hectic and busy lifestyle.

You also realize that eating clean can be incredibly delicious and tasty.

Now it's time for you to take action.

Get off the sidelines and get in the clean eating game. Your mental and physical health will benefit. You will trade chronic fatigue, disease and a host of negative health conditions for limitless energy, overall body health and fewer trips to the doctor. Isn't that something you deserve?

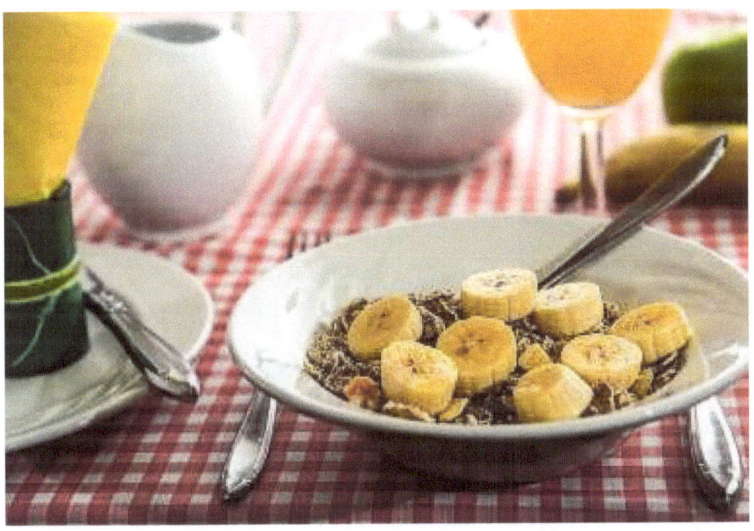

Other Relevant Books by This Author

If you would like to read more relevant books about this topic, here is a list of the CreateSpace links, titles and descriptions from this author:

https://www.createspace.com/6829717

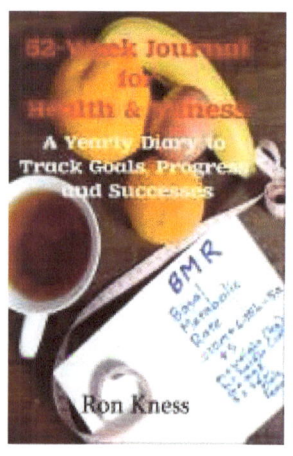

52-Week Journal for Health & Fitness: A Yearly Diary to Track Goals, Progress and Successes

By now, almost everyone has heard of journaling but you aren't sure why it is so beneficial or how to get started. Journaling is similar to keeping a diary, but it can be kept with specific self-help goals in mind such as this journal, like weight loss, hydration, health, exercise and fitness.

If your goal for the new year is to get healthier and live the healthy lifestyle, then this is the journal to record your goals, progress and successes.

Besides information on journaling and some history behind it, you'll find the following pages to write:
- Health and Fitness Goals
- Exercise and Fitness Goals
- Weeks 0-13 Measurements Chart
- Notes
- Weekly Planning 1-13
- Weeks 14-26 Measurements Chart
- Notes

- Weekly Planning 14 - 26
- Weeks 27 - 39 Measurements Chart
- Notes
- Weekly Planning 27 - 39
- Weeks 40-52 Measurements Chart
- Notes
- Weekly Planning 40 - 52

One benefit of journaling is that what gets recorded usually has a higher chance of getting done.

Get your copy today and start journaling for a better tomorrow!

https://www.createspace.com/6853248

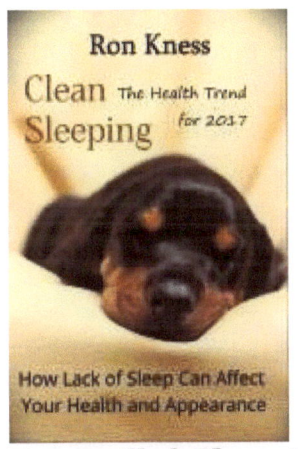

Clean Sleeping - The Health Trend for 2017: How Lack of Sleep Can Affect Your Health and Appearance

We want to be more energetic the next day . We also want to be more productive . And we want to get more sleep and of a better quality!

We can achieve ALL of these goals with the newest release from Ron Kness called *Clean Sleeping - The Health Trend For 2017*. Based on these exciting teachings, you will learn about all the dramatic benefits of restful sleep and eating foods that help people sleep better.

This book is built around a very clear, concept: feel well rested.

It's not just about ways to get the maximum amount of restorative sleep. Having great sleeping habits is linked to eating healthy. This is because some foods are more conducive to sleeping well than others

In this book, we look at all of the ways you can improve your own sleeping habits, starting with calming the mind. This book will also look at the many other steps that can be taken to support this goal, from doing meditation before retiring for the night to taking a warm bath scented with an essential oil and listening to soft music. Even the choices you make about healthy eating and creating sleep-inducing bedroom environment can have an impact on your sleeping habits.

In ***Clean Sleeping - The Health Trend For 2017***, we'll cover all the bases, giving you everything you need to know to get the maximum amount of quality sleep each night. It is the most important thing you can do for your overall physical and mental health.

The good news is that getting a good night's rest is totally doable ... we show you how!

https://www.createspace.com/6435460

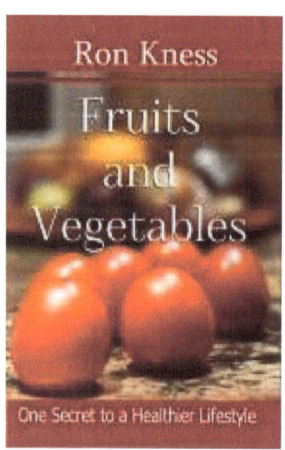

Fruits and Vegetables: One Secret to a Healthier Lifestyle

The way the human body processes food has not changed for thousands of years, however, our predominant food supply has. With the advent of modern agricultural and food processing methods, we have seen a lock-and-step increase in heart disease, cancer and other dangerous and deadly conditions.

That is because modern-day food is unfortunately highly processed. Salt and refined sugar, monosodium glutamate (MSG) and trans fats, preservatives, steroids and man-made chemicals are intentionally injected into most of the food you eat.

This is not done to make you healthier. It is simply done to make the food longer on store shelves, taste better, and to produce as addictive a product as possible (so that you will buy more of it).

Fresh vegetables and fruits (not fried or slathered in unhealthy dressing) have naturally healthy levels of the nutrients, minerals and vitamins your body needs. They do not contain the processed sugar, insanely high levels of salt, steroids, preservatives and other nutritionally bankrupt chemicals found in processed food.

Unfortunately, the fruits and vegetables that human beings once used to eat in abundance are now lacking in most diets. Your body still craves the same nutrition requirements it did when your ancestors were eating healthy foods.

However, if you continue to reward your hunger with too much unhealthy processed food, and not enough healthy fruits and vegetables, poor health and debilitating medical conditions will be your reward.

The fact that you are a product of nature, and fruits and vegetables are natural food sources, reveals why they are so important as a part of your healthy diet plan.

Another important aspect of swapping out processed foods for vegetables and fruits has to do with how much you weigh. If you find it hard to lose weight and maintain a slim, trim, sexy figure, your diet is probably to blame.

In this book, we explore the fruits and vegetables you should be eating, how much of each you should be eating each day and share some tips on how to increase your fruit and vegetable consumption. Change your diet today and enjoy good health tomorrow and beyond!

About the Author

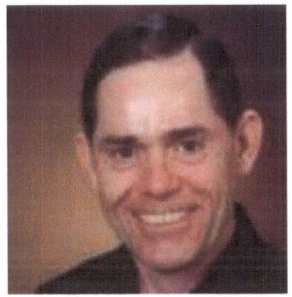

I have published over 125 books on Amazon for Kindle, CreateSpace and other publishing platforms.

While most of my books are on health and fitness in general, as I age (now 65) at the time of this writing) my topics of interest are geared toward aging baby boomers and older.

Besides my own writing, I also ghostwrite ebooks, books, reports, articles, blogs and do Kindle conversions for clients on a variety of topics.

Today my wife and I are retired from our careers and live in Gold Canyon, AZ. I now write as a retirement business where you'll find me happily sitting in my office typing away on my laptop as I work on my next book or ghostwriting project . . . that is if we are not traveling on a cruise ship - our new-found mode of travel.

www.ingramcontent.com/pod-product-compliance
Lightning Source LLC
Chambersburg PA
CBHW050831290526
45792CB00001B/346